Radiant Skin - Acne Treatment Book

Proven Acne Treatments, Remedies & Acne Diet To Cure Cystic & Hormonal Acne For Radiant Skin Fast. BONUS Acne Scar Treatments Chapter!

by Aimee Blake
© Copyright 2017

Copyright © 2017 Aimee Blake All rights reserved.
ISBN-13: 978-1976378997
ISBN-10:1976378990

All rights reserved. No part of this publication may be reproduced, distributed, or transmitted in any form or by any means, including photocopying, recording, or other electronic or mechanical methods, without the prior written permission of the publisher, except in the case of brief quotations embodied in reviews and certain other non-commercial uses permitted by copyright law.

While all attempts have been made to verify the information provided in this publication, neither the author, nor the publisher assumes any responsibility for errors, omissions, or contrary interpretations on the subject matter herein. This book is for entertainment purposes only. The views expressed are those of the author alone, and should not be taken as expert instruction or commands.

The reader is responsible for his or her own actions. A few affiliate links are included throughout this book. All products recommended have been personally used and tested by the author. Reader or purchaser are advised to do their own research before making any purchase online.

Adherence to all applicable laws and regulations, including international, federal, state, and local governing professional licensing, business practices, advertising, and all other aspects of doing business in the US, Canada, Australia or any other jurisdiction is the sole responsibility of the reader or purchaser.

Neither the author nor the publisher assumes any responsibility or liability whatsoever on the behalf of the purchaser or reader of these materials. Any perceived slight of any individual or organization is purely unintentional.

Table of Contents

Free Gift 1

Introduction 2

Causes of Acne 8

    Inflammation 8

    Hormones 11

    Gut Health 12

    Adult Acne 14

    Medications 15

    Cosmetics 16

    Other Causes 17

    Acne Journal 18

    Personal Action Plan 19

Internal Health 21

    Healing Vitamins 21

    Hydration 25

pH Balance   28

Apple Cider Vinegar (ACV)   30

Green Juices   32

Acne Free Diet 37

Food Sensitivity & Allergies   41

Internal Health Action Plan   44

External Health   47

Facial Cleansers to Reduce Acne   47

Moisturizers & Serums For Acne-Prone Skin   54

Spot Treatments for Acne Outbreaks   59

Makeup & Cosmetics   64

Skin Care Action Plan   69

Emotional & Physical Health   71

The Truth About Stress & Acne 71

Exercise, Acne & You   76

Time To Sweat It Out 81

Emotional & Physical Health Action Plan 86

Natural Acne Remedies 88

Turmeric Facial Mask 90

Soothing Oatmeal Facial 91

Yogurt & Yeast Mask (Oily Skin Only) 92

Grape Facial Cleanser 93

Healing Honey Mask 93

Baking Soda Facial 94

Apple Cider Vinegar 95

Tea Tree Oil 96

Purifying Egg White Mask 97

Lemon Juice 97

Light Therapy 99

Natural Remedies Action Plan 102

Prescription Acne Treatments 104

10 Most Frequently Used Acne Medications   105

Prescription Acne Action Plan   113

A Step By Step Radiant Skin Action Plan 114

Bonus - Acne Scar Treatments   124

Types of Acne Scars   124

Natural Scar Treatments   127

Lemon Juice   127

Potato Juice   130

Tomato Pulp   130

Aloe Vera   132

Essential Oils   132

Cucumber   135

Green Papaya   136

Orange Peels   137

Fenugreek Extract   137

Neem Leaves   138

Egg Whites 139

Turmeric 140

Honey 141

Fuller's Earth 141

Curds 142

Coconut Water 143

Sandalwood 143

Natural Skin Exfoliants 144

Choosing Acne Scar Treatment Products 149

Sunscreen 149

Silicone gels, sheets, dressings, and bandages 151

Ingredients to Look Out For In Over the Counter Products 151

Professional Scar Removal Treatments 157

Microdermabrasion 158

Chemical Peels 158

Skin Needling   159

Injectable Fillers   160

Ablative Resurfacing 160

Non Ablative Resurfacing 161

Factional CO2 Resurfacing   162

Combination Treatments   163

Surgery   163

Tissue Fillers   164

Corticosteroid Injections   164

Radio Frequency (RF) Treatments 166

Acne Scar Tips and Tricks   167

Free Gift 171

Other Books By Aimee 172

About The Author 174

Free Gift

Get your FREE "Radiant Skin - Beat Acne Checklist"

Print out this DAILY checklist with step by step instructions on what you should do in the morning, afternoon and night to help you beat acne!

Get your FREE "Acne Checklist" at:

Goo.gl/b9n1mw

Introduction

This acne treatment book contains proven strategies and step by step instructions on how to prevent and overcome adult acne - especially if you're experiencing cystic acne and hormonal acne.

Hi, I'm Aimee. Acne is a problem I've battled with for many years, so I know first hand the pain and embarrassment it causes.

I've been to countless doctors, dermatologist and skin specialists…
only to be prescribed oral medication and harsh topical creams that left my face looking red and scaly.

As the years went by, I began to look older than my age and my skin worsened to dry red painful skin.

After months of crying and feeling sorry for myself - I began to feel angry.

I had enough.

It was time to stop listening to all these so called "experts" and take matters into my own hands.

In this book, you're going to skip endless hours of research and find tested solutions on:
- How to get rid of acne fast
- Natural acne remedies that work
- Safe, natural and highly effective acne products

- And the anti aging and weight loss tips I discovered along the way!

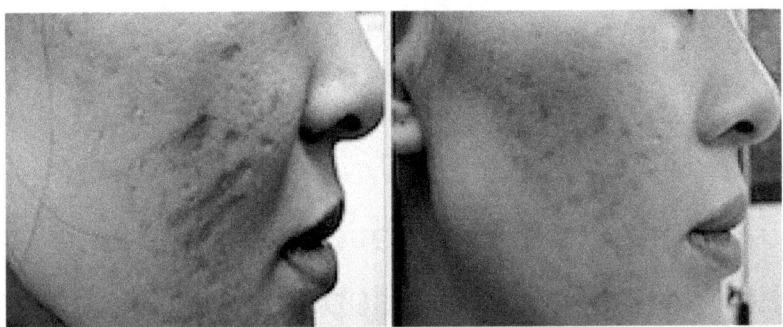

Acne left me with scarring but it has improved over the years. You'll get a bonus on how to get rid of acne scars too as a thank you for purchasing this book!

"Acne is much more than skin deep, it is the first sign of health problems to come"

Through research, I discovered that the causes of acne was multi-factorial and that it was a combination of internal and external health issues.

Acne is your body's way of telling you that there is inflammation, unbalanced hormones, toxin buildup and/or your digestive system is not functioning properly.

One of the reasons could be diet related like food sensitivity. For example, I removing gluten and wheat from my diet cleared up my skin significantly. This may or may not apply to you.

The purpose of this book is to show you the REAL causes of acne, how it can be eliminated and yes ... even cured through simple and easy to follow steps.

The recommendations you're about to read are from personal testing, trial and error and validated on scientific evidence.

Since you are your own unique self, I'll provide you with only the proven options and action plans to help you implement these methods.

Once you understand exactly what acne is, what causes and how to treat it with the strategies shown in this book - you too can enjoy blemish free, beautiful skin that mother nature intended for you to have.

Throughout this book, you will see a * **personal tip** to mark that the information is important and worth paying attention to.

Ready? Let's dive in.

Causes of Acne

Over the past decade, advancements in medicine and technology has increased our understanding of acne. We now know that there are **two primary causes for acne:** inflammation and hormones.

Here's a general overview of the main causes of acne:

Inflammation
Many researchers believe that inflammation in the skin is the trigger that starts the acne formation process.

To understand skin inflammation, you need a quick understanding of the skin's surface, the hair follicles and role of sebum production.

Here's how it works: your skin produces its own oil, called sebum.

The purpose of sebum is to oil your hair shaft and spread out over the top of the skin, sealing in moisture so that your skin stays healthy, youthful and wrinkle free.

Acne forms when there is an overproduction of sebum and when the natural oils of your skin become clogged in the pore.

If this occurs under the skin, a whitehead forms. If it occurs at the surface of the skin, it is known as a blackhead.

Inflammation and even infection occurs when these clogged pores become more and more enlarged over time, allowing bacteria to get deeper into the skin.

However there are internal sources of inflammation that have a direct connection to acne, these include:
- Gut issue and a lack of good bacteria
- Sensitivity and allergy to certain foods (wheat or gluten)
- Smoking and alcohol
- Stress (both emotional and physical)
- Lack of sleep (adults require 7-9 hours for body repair)

- Unhealthy diet (excessive fried and sugary foods)
- Imbalance of omega 3 and 6 fatty acids (consumed from the diet and referred as "essential fatty acids")
- Overconsumption of trans-fats (cookies, muffins, pies and cakes are examples of foods that may contain trans fat)
- Infections (bacteria can cause infection in your skin)

Hormones

The first experience that most people have with acne is during puberty, which brings us to the next cause of acne: hormones.

"All acne is to some degree hormonal"

Like inflammation, hormones accelerate sebum and keratin production, skin cell growth and regulate inflammatory response in the skin.

These hormones react with the skin to form dihydrotestosterone (DHT) - a hormonal by product of testosterone that occurs naturally in men and women which makes the sebaceous glands increase in size.

This results in an overproduction of sebum, plugs the hair follicles and eventually leads to the development of acne.

Gut Health
The human digestive track is inhabited by a large number of bacteria. Most of

which resides in the colon, with the stomach and small intestine being relatively sterile.

For the most part we coexist with these bacteria in a mutually beneficial relationship so they are good bacteria.

When you have bacteria disturbances in your gut, it results in digestive problems like bloating, constipation, nutrient loss, increase in stress and emotional issues.

The result of this ongoing struggle can influence the health of your hormones and health of your skin.

Bacterial imbalance in the gut can affect the bacteria on your skin, and taking probiotics has shown an increase in omega-3 levels in the blood resulting in a decrease in acne.

Adult Acne

For adults still suffering from acne, an excessive production or sensitivity to the body's hormones can exacerbate acne.

If both your male and female hormones are out of balanced, then this too can cause sebum production to increase and breakouts to happen.

For example women can experience an increase in estrogen during menstruation, the changes in estrogen during her monthly cycle will affect the severity of acne.

Medications

Some types of medicine can aggravate acne breakouts. For example, oral corticosteroids can cause acne by increasing yeast within the hair follicle.

Contraception like Depo Provera injections, Implanon or oral contraceptions which reduce the circulating sex hormone binding globulin (SHBG) can sometimes (not always) aggravate acne in women.

Lastly anabolic steroids like stanzolol, danazol etc can cause severe acne. The use of drugs may mess with your hormonal balance so consider talking to your doctor to determine if acne is a potential side effect of your medication.

Cosmetics

Acne Cosmetica is a term for cosmetics and skincare products that worsen acne. Heavy makeup or leaving makeup on can aggravate acne, as it allows the skin's natural oils to build up and potentially clog the pores.

Choose make up that is noncomedogenic (which means it does not contain ingredients that clog the pores) and clean your makeup applicators or brushes regularly as they may contain bacteria that is causing acne.

In an upcoming chapter, I'll cover what you should look out for in make-up and make specific cosmetic recommendations that are suitable for acne prone skin.

Other Causes

Other lifestyle factors can aggravate acne or cause breakouts. For example, oral contraceptives, may reduce acne breakouts in some individuals but increase them in others.

A busy stress and work lifestyle may cause an imbalance in your hormones and result in acne.

A bacteria that occurs naturally in hair follicles can cause problems if too much of it accumulates; but, again, some people are simply more sensitive to this reaction than others.

Acne Journal

Because every individual is different, the best way to determine what factors affects your acne is to keep a journal.

I know life can get busy but you only need to journal for 2 weeks to help identify the causes and triggers in your acne breakouts.

Keep note of what medications you're taking, what makeup you're wearing, how often you washed your face and with what cleanser – and, of course, whether or not you are currently experiencing a breakout.

Making connections regarding your acne and its potential causes is the first step toward eliminating it before resorting to acne treatments.

Personal Action Plan
Keep a journal that tracks the following things to help determine whether your unique acne triggers are:
- acne breakouts *(where they occur, how severe, and how long they last)*
- your diet *(write down what you ate for breakfast, lunch and dinner)*
- herbal or prescription medications you take *(including contraceptives and supplements)*
- your skin care regimen every day (changes in products or makeup)
- any other factors you think are significant, or may play a role (stress at work or arguments with loved ones)

Internal Health

Because acne is such a visible, surface ailment, it is easy to overlook the role that your overall internal health may play. Often, illness and imbalances inside your body is reflected on the skin.

Skin tone, texture and clarity can be a direct result of your diet. So the first step towards clear skin is to address the current condition of your internal health of your body.

Healing Vitamins

There are several vitamins and minerals that are important in preventing the development of acne, however none so important as Vitamin A and B Vitamins.

Vitamin A and B should be ideally absorbed through food and diet. However for convenience, consuming these 2 vitamins via supplements I was able to reduce inflammation of the skin.

Vitamin A

Vitamin A allows oil that flows from your glands and into the pores of your skin to function in a normal and healthy manner (aka it reduces sebum production that can clog pores and irritate the skin).

Vitamin A is a powerful antioxidant and important in achieving healthy skin, a deficiency of this vitamin can cause acne. Recommended dosage: take approximately 10,000 IU of vitamin A daily. Pregnant women should not take anymore than 5000 IU daily.

B Vitamins

B Vitamins are not only essential for general health and well being but also important in promoting healthy skin cells.

B vitamins cannot be stored by the body and have to be consumed regularly in the diet or through supplements.

When your skin is deficient in B vitamins, it can result in redness, irritation, dermatitis, pigmentation and acne.

Thiamine (B1) is an antioxidant which enhances circulation and assists in digestion. Recommended dosage is to get 300 mg of vitamin B1 taken every day, morning, day and night.

Riboflavin (B2) is essential for healthy skin, hair and nails. Just being deficient in vitamin b2 alone can be a symptom of acne. Recommended dosage required to help clear up acne is 300 mgs of vitamin b2, taken every day, morning, day and night.

Niacin (B3) improves skin circulation and helps to pull toxins out of your system faster. Although you can take B3 as a supplement, niacin or niacinimide when applied topically is one of the *most ground breaking discoveries* of the B's I have found for treating acne.

I learnt this from a skin doctor who created a range of skin medicines (also known as cosmeceuticals) and it works by enhancing local breakdown of androgens *(I will cover this in more detail in chapter 3).*

Vitamin B5 is also an important vitamin, helping to reduce stress and supporting good adrenal function.

Pyridoxine, or vitamin B6, supports the immune system and the production of antibodies.

Although I have recommended specific dosages, I have found that "B Vitamin Complex" ordered online or at your local drug store/chemist is suffice.

Hydration

Hydration or water is the first, and most important, part of maintaining healthy skin. Your body loses moisture constantly – when you sweat, cry and even breathe.

If you don't take in at least as much water as you lose, then you can quickly become dehydrated.

When you're dehydrated, it causes the skin to dry and dead skin cells to build up on the skin. These dead skin cells can clog pores, indirectly contributing to your acne breakouts.

Also, the glands that produce sebum may respond to dry skin by producing excess oil, which can increase the number of clogged pores.

So, how much water do you need to drink for optimum skin health?

According to the Mayo Clinic and The Institute of Medicine, a healthy intake for women is roughly 9 cups of water per day and for men, 13 cups of water per day.

This can include fruit juices, teas, smoothies and other beverages *(provided they don't have added sugar)* so you don't have to haul around a huge jug of water all day to stay properly hydrated.

Remember: Although all liquids count towards your daily hydration total, drinking clean pure water is always best as it not only provides your body with moisture but it also detoxes it.

Lastly, don't overdo it with drinking water. Too much water can cause an imbalance in your electrolyte levels which are crucial for keeping your body's fluid levels balanced.

pH Balance

Another key acne trigger is the overall pH balance of your body and skin. The balance of alkaline and acid in your body can vary greatly, ranging from one to fourteen.

Anything below 7 is acidic; anything above is alkaline. Skin is usually healthiest when it stays within the range of 4 and 6.5.

This ideal balance helps skin cells multiply and function properly, as well as kill off excess bacteria which can contribute to acne outbreaks.

The most frequent question asked is how do you know your internal body is pH balanced?

There are pH test strips that you can buy on Amazon to test your body's pH levels for alkaline and acid levels using Saliva and urine.

Once you've tested on your pH levels, pay attention to what you eat and what you put on your skin to help keep your pH levels in check.

For instance, one study indicated that eating foods high in monounsaturated fats led to a 6% increase in participants' pH levels.

Conversely, another study showed that applying a vitamin A-rich serum to the skin reduced the level of pH by 3 percent.

Additionally, twice-daily cleansing with a product that is pH-balanced is extremely important as is using a pH balanced *(but not oily)* moisturizer.

Apple Cider Vinegar (ACV)

Besides the skin, alkalizing your body's internal system can help you remove unwanted toxins.

Your blood needs to be slightly alkaline to keep you healthy, and consuming some apple cider vinegar can help you achieve that goal.

In fact, societies worldwide have long accepted the healing properties of apple cider vinegar, from the Greek physician Hippocrates to Japan's famous Samurai warriors.

Apple cider vinegar (ACV) contains acetic acid, an important element in balancing the body's pH and many other health benefits.

* **Personal tip:** I use Bragg's ACV to balance my overall pH levels by following this simple recipe. Add two tablespoons of apple cider vinegar to 8-16 ounces of plain, filtered water and drink every day.

Warning: Your body may purge all the toxins to your skin's surface so you might experience more acne and look worse in the first week before you look better.

However as the weeks go by and as your body becomes more alkaline, you will notice a reduction in acne especially for those who have cystic acne.

Green Juices

Green juices and smoothies that are made with vegetables and fruit are also a great way to balance your body's pH by alkalizing your internal systems.

The green juices I make tend to have 80% greens and 20% fruit - it's better for my skin and diet *(as sugar in fruit makes you more hungry!)*.

Smoothies and shakes made with fresh green juices provide an alkalizing effect on the body, and they provide countless other health benefits too.

Mixing up a green vegetable/leaf and some fruit as a smoothie for breakfast or healthy snack will help brighten your skin and improve overall physical health.

Now there are hundreds of green juices available online but if you're busy and like simple recipes that are easy to prepare.

Below are three green smoothies I drank while battling my acne - all you need to do is prep the fruit and blend until smooth.

Green-colada Super Shake

Ingredients:
- 4 cups baby spinach leaves
- ½ avocado (scooped out and pitted)
- 1 cucumber
- 2 squeezed grapefruits (use juice only)
- 1 medium coconut (use meat only)
- Several ice cubes

Green Vanilla-Lime Power Shake

Ingredients:
- 1 cup fresh baby spinach leaves (or Kale leaves)
- 2 tbsp fresh lime juice
- 2 teaspoons raw honey
- ½ fresh banana
- ½ cup almond milk

- A dash of vanilla extract
- 1 cup of ice

Kiwi-Spinach Smoothie

Ingredients:
- 2 peeled kiwis (gold or green kiwi)
- 1 cup spinach leaves
- ½ banana
- ½ cup apple juice
- Several ice cubes

* **Personal tip:** When I'm working long hours without a blender or nearby grocery, I carry along a tub of "Organifi" powder.

I am in love with this drink because you can get all your healthy superfoods in one drink without any blending or juicing.

The health benefits of Organifi are amazing:
- If you don't have time or if you're traveling, you can literally grab a green juice on the go!
- Incredible energy, focus and mental clarity which helps you become more productive throughout the day
- Supports internal health as mentioned throughout this chapter with electrolytes in coconut water
- Reduces stress by balancing hormones already within normal range and reduces yourself from frustrations
- Detoxifies your body by flushing out toxins
- Healthy and radiant skin from the nutrients and minerals in the

ingredients by promoting healthy hair, skin and nails.

Acne Free Diet

The standard American or western diet consists primarily of processed foods which are woefully deficient in the basic micro nutrients required to create both hormones and healthy skin.

Therefore your existing diet may be nutritionally deprived and highly susceptible in developing severe acne.

For the most part, a diet that promotes blemish free skin is a common sense diet:
- plenty of fruits and vegetables
- quality fats like coconut oil
- Lean protein

- olive oil and avocado
- minus highly processed foods.

A few nutrients are known to be good for the skin. Vitamin A is actually the main ingredient in Accutane, as it's key to regulating the cycles of healthy skin. Other minerals are known to be helpful too.

Foods rich in Vitamin A are:
- Sweet potato
- Carrots
- Kale
- Squash
- Cos & Romaine Lettuce
- Dried Apricots
- Sweet peppers
- Salmon/Tuna

Zinc is believed to help reduce acne by inhibiting the growth of acne-causing bacteria. Foods high in Zinc are:
- Lamb
- Pumpkin seeds
- Grass fed beef
- Chick peas
- Cashews
- Mushrooms
- Spinach
- Chicken

Vitamin C and vitamin E help to soothe the skin and prevent inflammation. Foods high in Vitamin C are:
- Oranges
- Red peppers
- Kale
- Brussels sprouts
- Broccoli

- Strawberries
- Guava
- Kiwi

Omega-3 fatty acids (also available in supplements) are also recommended, because they promote the growth of new skin cells.

These healthy fatty acids can be found in a variety of foods, including avocados, sunflower seeds and fish.

It's ideal to get these nutrients by including them in your diet however a good dietary supplement can also provide the same benefits for your skin.

However having a daily green drink like Organifi will definitely provide essential vitamins and nutrients to your skin and complement the acne diet to reduce inflammation.

Oganifi Ingredients: organic Moringa, chlorella, mint, spirulina, ashwagandha, beets, wheatgrass, turmeric, lemon and coconut water

Food Sensitivity & Allergies

After conducting some research, studies show people who had Irritable Bowel Syndrome (IBS) also had some degree of inflammation to the gut.

As discussed before, inflammation is one of the main causes and triggers of acne.

In a test done by Italian scientists at the University Hospital of Palermo, they put 160 IBS patients on an elimination diet of wheat, all forms of dairy products, caged eggs, chocolate and tomatoes.

After 4 weeks on this elimination diet, they found that 70 (43%) of the patients improved. Then they challenged those 40 people with wheat and cow's milk.

Out of those 40 people, 30 had a negative reaction to both wheat and cow's milk, 6 to cow's milk alone and 4 to wheat alone.

From that study, you can surmise that the common food problems that caused inflammation were from: milk and wheat.

If you happen to have IBS, digestive problems or regular occurrences of constipation, perhaps its time to eliminate dairy and wheat from your diet.

In terms of eggs, they are a great source of protein and omega 3 fats which protects against heart disease and some inflammatory diseases.

So I wouldn't rule out eggs entirely, however swapping caged eggs for free range eggs may make a difference to your acne.

* **Personal tip:** The first thing I did was cut out wheat and dairy products from my diet and the results have been nothing but spectacular.

It resulted in a trimmer waist line, 10 pounds in weight loss and reduction of acne breakouts.

Consider me a believer. That alone was enough for me to stick to a gluten free and diary free diet permanently.

Internal Health Action Plan
1. Take vitamin A, B vitamin complex and probiotics for skin cell renewal and good gut health.
2. Maintain proper hydration (~9 cups of liquid for women and ~13 for men)
3. A healthy body is slightly alkaline measuring approximately 7.4. You can purchase Alkaline PH Tests from Amazon to determine if you're too acidic.

4. If you are, add 1 tablespoon of apple cider vinegar (with mother i.e. cloudy apple cider vinegar) into 8 cups of water and drink daily until you notice an improvement. If the taste bothers you, mix in raw honey or some apple juice.
5. Replace your morning coffee with a green smoothie like Organifi and feel the difference it makes to your energy levels and skin.
6. Eat a common sense nutritious diet to reduce acne triggers in your foods and increase helpful nutrients. This includes eating fruits, veggies, fish or lean protein to ensure a diet high in zinc, vitamin E, vitamin A and Omega 3 fatty acids.

7. Consider cutting out wheat and dairy for 2 weeks *(try almond milk instead)* add this to your acne journal and see if you notice a difference in your acne outbreak.

External Health

Now that we've discussed the relationship between your body's internal health and acne, let's talk about the importance of external skin care.

Since acne forms at the surface of your skin, what you put on it and how you treat it can have a major impact on acne breakouts.

One of the most important things you can do is create a healthy and consistent skin care regime that meets your lifestyle and skin care needs.

Facial Cleansers to Reduce Acne

Any great skin care regimen for acne reduction should begin with a great cleanser (and they are often have few ingredients).

Harsh soaps and a rough scrubbing will only result in inflamed skin that can actually increase acne.

The right cleanser for acne-prone skin doesn't have to come with a prescription, it can be found right on the shelf at your local drug store or super market.

No matter where you get your facial cleanser, there are a few important things to look for.

First, you should select a cleanser that is gentle on your skin and pH balanced.

This means non-abrasive, nor rough and exfoliating cleansers.

Although regular, gentle exfoliating is recommended for acne-prone skin, too much can inflame sensitive areas.

Your chosen cleanser should be soap free, foam free, alcohol free and paraben free (limit any harsh chemicals).

Look for a cleanser that is specifically formulated for your skin type, be it dry, oil or combination skin.

When shopping for acne cleansers, you'll notice that some of them contain extra acne fighters. These might include benzoyl peroxide or salicylic acid.

While these acne cleansers can be effective to alleviate the symptoms *(we'll go into more detail later)*, they can also have a drying effect on skin.

Plus, if you're using an additional product with these ingredients, like a spot treatment or lotion, using cleansers with these active ingredients will only irritate the skin.

* **Personal Tip:** I use "Cetaphil Gentle Cleanser" and a micro fibre cloth to aid in my face cleansing.

This cleanser is gentle on the skin, maintains your skin's PH level and the micro fibre cloth can wipe away excess dirt and grime.

Benefits of Toner for Reducing Acne

Although facial toners are not as common in skin-care regimes as they used to be, the right toner can have many benefits when it comes to reducing acne.

Most importantly, toners help balance the pH level of your skin.

As we mentioned previously, a balanced pH level of between 4 and 6.5 is the key to maintaining vibrant, clear skin and discouraging breakouts.

Toners work to remove toxins that your cleanser may have missed, for overall cleaner skin. They also help shrink and tighten pores making your face look firmer.

This can reduce acne outbreaks, as smaller pores are less likely to become clogged by oil or dead skin cells. For many people suffering from acne, the addition of toner to their skin care regimen comes as a pleasant surprise.

 * **Personal tip:** I made my own facial toner using Apple Cider Vinegar (ACV). Yep, ACV again is not only good internally but has antibacterial and antiseptic properties to help balance out your skin.

Remember, you need to have pH-balanced skin because without it, your skin will... pardon my language, will look like shit. It will look dull and lifeless.

ACV has a pH of 3 and when diluted, the acidity from the toner helps bring your skin's pH back to its normal levels.

Recipe: Easy Apple Cider Vinegar Toner

Ingredients:
- 1/2 c. distilled or filtered water
- 1/2 Tbsp apple cider vinegar (with mother)
- Instructions:
- Mix together in a small bottle.
- Store in the fridge.
- Should keep up to 2 weeks.

Toner Products

If you prefer to buy your own toners or don't like the smell of ACV, I recommend Now Foods, Purifying Toner, Vitamin C & Acai Berry from herb.com.

You can purchase the above toner from iherb.com and get 5% off which only costs $6.88 at the time of writing!

Moisturizers & Serums For Acne-Prone Skin

Your skin's natural moisture is great, but an overproduction of those natural oils isn't.

In fact, since that oil is clogging your pores and causing inflammation, you'll need to wash carefully without stripping out your skin.

And afterwards, you'll need to replace that moisture with something that doesn't irritate your acne. But how do you find a moisturizer or serum for your acne-prone skin that won't make the problem worse?

Ok, remember in chapter 3 I mentioned B vitamins and how I discovered a break through for beating acne was Niacin

(B3)? Well niacinimide, also known as vitamin B3 plays an important role in cellular energy production.

It has anti-inflammatory properties, which makes it effective for treating acne and anti aging benefits for more mature skin *(who doesn't want to look younger?)*

There's some evidence that suggests niacin stimulates cells in the dermis to produce more collagen, a protein that supports skin and gives it its youthful firmness.

That's a good thing since collagen levels decline with age, and loss of collagen is a major cause of wrinkles and saggy skin.

So if you have adult acne especially with cystic acne, you're in luck as you can not only treat acne but aging skin!

In a randomly controlled study, 76 patients with moderate acne were treated using a 4% niacinimide gel vs a 1% clindamycin gel (a topical antibiotic).

After 8 weeks, 82% of patients who were treated with niacinimide reported successful results compared to those treated with clindamycin.

This research indicates that the anti-inflammatory activity of a 4% niacinimide serum or gel was effective in treating acne.

Even a topical formulation of niacinimide at higher concentration of up to 10% is stable, safe and well tolerated on the skin.

* **Personal tip:** I make my own Niacinimide serum at 5% strength - all of the ingredients can be purchased online via amazon or iherb.

The below recipe is simple and has kept my skin baby smooth and blemish free. Niacinimide powder comes in a fine white powder and dissolves easily in distilled water.

Recipe: Niacinimide Serum 5%
You will need a scale. Ingredients:
- 5% Niacinimide powder
- 2% Hyaluronic acid
- 93% Distilled Water

Instructions:

- Mix everything together until dissolved
- Store in a sterilized jar and refrigerate.
- Should keep up to 2 weeks.
- Apply the serum on a clean face at night before bed

Niacinimide Products

If you don't have a sterile environment and prefer to buy your own niacinimide serum, I recommend these 2 products:

1. Acnessential 4% Topical Niacinamide cream
2. Skin Daily Niacinamide Vitamin B3 Cream Serum 5%

I spent some time researching the best niacinimide serums and these two are the best on Amazon - they have high quality ingredients, positive reviews and are affordable.

Spot Treatments for Acne Outbreaks

If you tracked your acne breakouts with a journal, implemented the internal health action plan and the suggested skin care regime - that alone should stop acne in its tracks.

However there are times where you need to zap a zit fast and it is the only time I recommend using spot treatments.

Spot treatments are over-the-counter or prescription creams that work to break and dry up sebum in the treated area.

They can also help to stop acne outbreaks by slowing the growth of acne-causing bacteria or killing it altogether.

There are two primary ingredients in spot creams today – **benzoyl peroxide** and **salicylic acid.**

Benzoyl peroxide and salicylic acid are the most popular and effective ingredients included in acne spot treatments.

Benzoyl peroxide is generally accepted as the strongest and most effective treatment for acne that is available without a prescription.

It works by eliminating the bacteria that cause acne, clearing the clogged pores and allowing pimples to heal.

Spot treatments with benzoyl peroxide are available in different strengths, usually a 2.5%, 5% or 10% concentration.

When using benzoyl peroxide for the first time, it's best to start at the lower strengths, either a 2.5% or 5%.

If you don't notice a visible improvement after approximately four weeks, you can move to the stronger 10% benzoyl peroxide creams.

Salicylic acid is another spot treatment ingredient known for its effectiveness. This popular acne-fighting ingredient helps to heal acne by exfoliating the skin, unclogging pores and actually decreasing inflammation.

This is unusual among acne treatments, as most of them have an irritating effect on skin as it adjusts. Salicylic acid actually soothes the skin, which is perfect for already-irritated areas.

Acne spot treatments should not be used over the entire face; they are most effective as a complement to a regular skin regimen that is designed to fit your individual needs.

When using benzoyl peroxide or salicylic acid spot treatments, it's important to **start slow** and pay attention to any dryness.

Start by applying a thin film to the entire area of the break out or individual pimple once a day. Do not apply to thin delicate skin around the mouth, eyes or nostrils.

If the skin in that area doesn't become red or sore, apply treatment twice a day – in the morning and evening.

As noted above, the strength can eventually increase if dryness and irritation doesn't persist.

Spot Treatment Products
I have personally used Benzac Intenstive Spot treatment. After going through several products, this product not leave my skin looking scaly or red unlike other spot treatments.

Note: the higher the % strength doesn't mean it's better. It could strip your skin and cause severe irritation so stick with low doses at first and gradually increase strength as required.

Though I rarely use this anymore as my skin has cleared up, every now and then I use spot treatments.

If you're skin does not like benzoyl peroxide or salicylic acid, then you can use hydrogen peroxide or tree oil as a spot treatment

Makeup & Cosmetics

If you're a woman, you probably wore heavy makeup to cover up raging red pimples. However this stops your skin from breathing and end up clogging your pores.

Additionally touching your skin with fingers or using brushes to apply makeup can also pass on bacteria to your skin. Ensure that your hands and brushes are clean to reduce bacteria transfer.

Here's what to look for in makeup:
- Foundation: Look for water based formulas to avoid getting your clogged pores clogged up. Mineral and sunflower oil DO NOT penetrate into the pores so they are fine as ingredients. Be aware of products containing lanolin as they will clog up your pores.

- **Fragrances:** Fragrances may cause allergic reactions, some fragrances to avoid are musk, ambrette, and bergamot families. Look for fragrance-free products.
- **Eye shadows and blushes:** Mica is the most common mineral used in eyeshadows, blush and face powder because it creates shimmer. A small amount of mica is fine but test your skin to see if it reacts to it.
- Eye creams: avoid heavy eye creams or oily eye make-up removers as they are greasier and since they are near the forehead, cheeks and temples - the migration of oils can eventually cause acne.
- Lip products: lipsticks and lip gloss are greasy by nature, the greater the shine, the more potential for clogging

your skin pores. Stick to matte finished products instead of gloss.

Cosmetic Products

Whilst there are thousands of makeup and cosmetic options available, the products recommended below have been researched and tested personally.

I tend to err on the natural/organic side when it comes to makeup - however they tend to be much more expensive than makeup available over the counter.

1. Annmarie Skin Care Line

A fantastic line of mineral makeup however it does contain a small amount of mica. This doesn't have any reaction on my skin but if you have highly sensitive skin, opt for more natural and organic ingredients.

2. 100% Pure Tinted Moisturizer & Foundation

I love love this makeup company, they have an outstanding ingredients list with nourishing ingredients and so natural that you can eat the stuff!

3. ILIA Beauty

ILIA was founded on the ideology of simplicity and transparency. Their high quality ingredients are sourced from organic farmers around the world and manufactured in an organic certified lab. Their lab holds certifications with Gluten-Free, USDA Organic, and Leaping Bunny.

4. Gabriel Cosmetics

Gabriel Cosmetics started with a vision of natural beauty and has evolved with a philosophy that is translated through their NPA certified skincare as well as vegan.

Skin Care Action Plan

Create a healthy, acne-reducing skin care regimen for your skin and follow through in the morning and evening.

- Start with a simple micro-fiber cloth to clean your skin.
- Facial Cleansers - Find pH balanced cleanser that is gentle and non-abrasive for acne-prone skin i.e. Cetaphil Gentle Cleanser.
- Toner - Use a pH balancing toner as part of your regimen to help your skin maintain a pH that will inhibit acne

- Toner Moisturizer/Serums - A 4-5% niacinimide gel/serum applied at night is one of the main reasons why my skin cleared up so fast.
- Spot Treatments - Use spot treatments sparingly however opt for tea-tree oil first before going for Benzac spot treatment.
- Makeup - Opt for natural cosmetics that don't irritate your skin.

Emotional & Physical Health

Ever wondered if there was a connection to your emotional health, level of physical activity and acne outbreaks?

Well there is, scientists have discovered data linking acne in some way to both high levels of stress and working out.

The Truth About Stress & Acne

While there is surprisingly little research on stress and acne, one study showed that students had much more acne while under examination stress than during low-stress period.

During stress the brain releases a neurotransmitter called Substance P (SP).

SP can increase sebum production and cause inflammation in the skin, thus providing a direct link between stress and acne.

Noting your current stress levels in the acne journal discussed in Chapter 2 can help you make important connections when it comes to stress and your skin.

There are many different steps you can take to reduce the impacts of stress in your life.

Getting enough sleep and eating well are not only part of a healthy lifestyle, they can also give your body the power to combat the effects of stress.

Daily meditation or relaxation is perhaps the best way to reduce stress.

Studies have shown meditation and relaxation exercises are equally effective in reducing stress – meditation is better at reducing recurring negative thoughts, though.

So it doesn't matter which one you choose. The important thing is to do something regularly.

Working out is also a popular way to reduce stress and stay in shape.

In addition to the obvious physical benefits of exercise, the endorphins released during exercise work as nature's "chill pill", helping to relax muscles and give us a feeling of overall well-being.

Keeping track of your diet, getting enough sleep and working out regularly can be a lot to keep track of – especially on a busy schedule.

But these things really can make a difference when it comes to reducing acne outbreaks.

Below are a few popular smartphone apps and online resources that help you get the rest and relaxation.

1. Sleep Time – Alarm Clock
This smart sleep app helps you get the amount of rest you need every night. The phone's accelerometer can tell you how quickly you fall asleep, and when you enter each phase of sleep. When

it's time to wake, the app gently wakes you at an optimum time in your sleep cycle.

2. Relax & Rest Guided Meditations
Is an app offers help for those who want to relax, but aren't sure how. Several guided meditations are available ranging from 5 minutes to half an hour. They include Breath Awareness, Deep Rested Meditation and Whole Body Guided Relaxation. It's a great way to de-stress and relax wherever and whenever you need it.

3. Headspace
Headspace is a program that makes starting meditation easy and simple. Developed by a former Buddhist monk, the program delivers a different 10 minute meditation every day. It is the

easiest way to start and maintain your meditation habit.

The downside is that you have to pay either a monthly or yearly fee to access the meditations. They offer a 10-day meditation program for free – www.Getsomeheadspace.com

4. Calm

Calm is not an app but I have listed it here as a tool since it's completely free. You can can listen a 2, 10 or 20 minute guided relaxation at www.calm.com.

Exercise, Acne & You

Some say that exercising can make acne worse, while others say it helps to eliminate outbreaks. But which advice is true?

According to the National Institute of Arthritis and Musculoskeletal and Skin Diseases, or NIAMS, working out results in an increased flow of blood to the surface of your skin.

This increased blood flow helps to flush away impurities, as well as bringing a fresh supply of nutrients and oxygen to your skin.

I found that exercising DEFINITELY helps however there are *some* things that happen during and after workouts can cause acne to flare up.

Clothing that rubs against the skin can trap dirt and oils and make acne worse; this includes things like hats, sunglasses and other equipment.

Another big problem is what happens when you sweat.

Many people use a "workout" towel or inadvertently wipe their skin with their hands. These practices can transfer bacteria and oils to the skin, making acne worse.

The solution? incorporate exercise in your acne routine as it helps sweats out bacteria and toxins.

Here are some fantastic exercise apps that I LOVE that's free and doesn't require access to a gym:

1. Runtastic Results - Free App
This app doesn't require any equipment as each strength-training workouts is done with your bodyweight only. To start, you spell out what your goals are, and

they'll generate a personalized 12-week workout program.

When you start a workout, there are videos that demonstrate how to safely perform each exercise. It's a smart choice for beginners who want to build muscle, but aren't ready to pick up a weight yet.

2. Nike+ Training Club - Free App
This nifty app gives you access to a bunch of expert-led 15-45 minute workouts right from your phone. Professional athletes like Serena Williams and Kevin Hart make an appearance as well. The app talks you through exactly how to get the best of each workout, all while playing your favorite music in the background.

It's also aimed at both men and women with options to allow you to target any body part with beginner, intermediate and advanced exercises.

3. Freeletics Body Weights - Free App

As the name suggests, this app focuses on bodyweight-only exercises and is perfect if you don't have a gym membership. Before you choose one of the 10- to 30-minute workouts in this app, you have to complete a fitness test to assess your level.

The "virtual coach" will create a weekly training plan that's tailored to your abilities and goals. There are so many routines that are home-friendly and it will only show you workouts that can be done in two by two meters of space.

Get your exercise in however avoid touching your face in general, wear clean workout clothes, clean equipment after each use, use a fresh towel with every workout and shower immediately after a workout.

Time To Sweat It Out

When it comes to sweat and your skin, one thing is clear: working up a sweat opens your pores. But whether or not it is helpful in clearing acne is an area of debate.

Much of the debate depends on *how* you sweat; yes, according to some experts and sweat therapy enthusiasts, there is a *right* way to sweat.

And, when this "correct" sweat regimen is used, sweating can clear pores, remove impurities from the body and rid you of troublesome acne outbreaks.

This is also mean after you exercise or sweat, wash off the in the shower to remove those impurities.

One thing that everyone seems to agree on – when it comes to acne sufferers, dry heat is far better than moist heat, which can foster the growth of bacteria.

Saunas are recommended for those who want to open clogged pores and sweat away excess sebum and bacteria.

Any sauna will work well, often, they can be found at your local gym and if you're fortunate to live in a building that has one - use it!

Below are a few useful health tips for creating the perfect sauna regimen:

1. Don't overstay your welcome.
The recommended time for staying in a sauna is a maximum of 15-20 minutes. You can always cool down and then return to the sauna, but a stint of longer than 20 minutes can risk problems like heat stroke.

2. Only use a sauna regimen if you're in good health.
It's always best to be on the safe side. If you think you may be dehydrated or are suffering from a hangover, it's best to avoid the sauna.

For those who are pregnant, saunas are also warned against, as they can raise your core body temperature. If you are on medication or have any other significant health issues (like high blood pressure), it's best to speak with your doctor before beginning a sauna regimen.

3. Go into the sauna with clean, dry skin.
If you are wearing skin creams, acne treatments, lotions or make-up, be sure to clean your skin (particularly problem areas) before using the sauna.

When skin has make-up or other products on it, these can melt and mix with sweat in the sauna, causing them to clog pores further.

4. Use gentle massage.
Once you've started seating in the sauna, use a micro fibre cloth or

washcloth to gently massage your face and other problem areas. This helps the sweat more effectively break up the oil in the clogged pores before flushing it out.

5. Shower it off.
After your sauna treatment, it's important to take a shower to remove all of the sweat, oils, dirt and impurities that have been flushed out.

Most sauna enthusiasts suggest a warm shower that is later turned to cold before getting out, and that no soap be used to avoid contaminating freshly purified skin.

Your emotional and physical health can have a profound impact on your body's largest organ: the skin. Reducing stress and exercising as part of a healthy lifestyle can help your body maintain important balances.

A carefully planned sauna regimen can offer easy, natural and cost-effective relief to acne sufferers.

Incorporating these simple changes into your lifestyle can have long-lasting results in terms of acne reduction.

Emotional & Physical Health Action Plan

- Assess your current stress level. Download the recommended smart phone apps and make a point to relax and reduce your stress through meditation or exercise.

- Keep track of your stress levels in your acne journal to determine if there's a connection between stress and your outbreaks.
- Exercise regularly to reduce stress and improve the overall health of your body and skin. Make sure you shower straight away to remove dirt and sweat.
- Try a sauna regimen, following the helpful guidelines above.

Natural Acne Remedies

It would be ideal for you to try natural acne remedies first before you resort to any medications or prescription acne treatments.

Besides having to use over the counter spot treatments and a course of antibiotics *(never again! as it destroyed all the good bacteria in my gut),* I prefer natural acne remedies.

Most doctors will prescribe antibiotics or prescriptive medicine however the use of antibiotics strip **both** good and bacteria from your body and then your body can't defend all the other nasty bacteria.

Use antibiotics when extremely sick or ill, try to let your immune system fight it off with the use of water and vitamins first.

Besides maintaining internal health and external skin care, incorporate natural acne remedies once a week.

Now there are countless tried and true acne remedies either on the market or that can made right at home.

Many of these cost very little to try, and are found to be highly effective without any effects. Let's talk about a few of the most popular naturally-sourced acne remedies.

Turmeric Facial Mask

Turmeric is my all time favorite spice in battling acne - just applying turmeric paste reduced my inflamed pimples in less than a week!

This traditional Indian face turmeric mask is said to beautify skin and help clear acne.

To make this mask:
- Mix ½ cup chickpea flour with approximately two teaspoons of almond oil, sandalwood powder and turmeric powder (all of these ingredients can be found at an ethnic food market or an indian grocery store).

- Add enough water to create a paste, apply to skin and leave on for 5-10 minutes.
- Wipe excess paste off with your fingers and then rinse thoroughly with water.

Soothing Oatmeal Facial

Acne prone skin is often red, sore and irritated, and oatmeal facials are naturally soothing for overwrought skin.

To create this simple remedy:
- mix two teaspoons oatmeal with a pinch of baking soda
- add just enough water to make a paste
- Massage into your skin
- and let dry before rinsing thoroughly.

Yogurt & Yeast Mask (Oily Skin Only)

Since excess oil is a major trigger for acne, this oil-reducing mask can help clear and prevent acne breakouts.

To create this mask:
- mix one teaspoon of brewer's yeast
- with a bit of plain yogurt
- it should create a mix that is thin in consistently
- Apply directly to the face
- allow to set for around 20 minutes.
- rinse with warm water
- followed by a rinse with cold water to close the pores and soothe the skin.

Grape Facial Cleanser

Fresh grape extract makes an easy and 100% natural facial cleanser.

To make this cleanser:
- cut a handful of grapes in half
- rub the fruit over your face and neck.
- finish up with a cool water rinse
- and your skin will be naturally clean and beautiful.

Healing Honey Mask

Honey – that's right, *honey* – is a wonder of nature, with powerful antibacterial properties.

In fact, a honey mask can help to eliminate harmful, acne-causing bacteria that inhabit the pores.

To use this mask:
- first rinse your face with warm water
- apply *raw* organic honey directly to skin
- leave on for half an hour
- rinse with warm water
- followed by a cold water rinse to close pores.

Baking Soda Facial

Baking soda is known for having an incredible variety of uses, and helping to clear acne is one of them!

Baking soda soothes inflamed skin and exfoliates, helping to remove dead skin cells that can clog pores. It's easy, inexpensive and simple to prepare.

To make this facial:

- add a few teaspoons of baking soda in a bowl
- mix in warm water until it forms a paste
- and then apply to your skin
- leave it on for ten to fifteen minutes
- rinse with warm water
- followed up by a cold rinse.

Apple Cider Vinegar

Apple cider vinegar (with mother) is a popular natural acne remedy is antibacterial, helping to purify the skin and kill acne-causing bacteria.

Because it is such a powerful ingredient, you may want to start out with a 50/50 water and apple cider vinegar mixture.

You can always mix a stronger solution later on.

Using a cotton ball or cotton swab, apply it directly to your skin. You can leave it on, or rinse it off after a few minutes.

Tea Tree Oil

This essential oil is a potent natural remedy, and acts as an antibacterial agent when applied to the skin.

After mixing a small amount of tea tree oil with an equal portion of water, apply it with a cotton ball.

No need to rinse – this natural solution can be left on all day, even under make-up.

Purifying Egg White Mask

It may seem surprising, but plain egg whites make an amazing mask that can work wonders for acne prone skin.

In fact, an egg white mask works to draw out impurities, reduce pore size and minimize oil.

After separating the yolk and egg white, apply the egg white directly to your skin.

You can leave this mixture on for up to an hour before rinsing off with plain water.

Lemon Juice

One hundred percent natural lemon juice is both antibacterial and astringent, killing acne-causing bacteria and minimizing pores.

Although the best way is to use fresh-squeezed lemon juice, bottled lemon juice will also work.

Apply to your skin with a cotton ball. You can leave it on for up to an hour prior to rinsing.

These are several of the best known and most effective natural remedies for clearing and preventing acne.

They are all inexpensive and chemical free, so they're healthy for you and your skin. Try one or try them all, and find out which natural remedies can help you control your acne.

Light Therapy

Light therapies is not something you can whip up in your kitchen however it's worth mentioning as it is technically a natural acne treatment.

It is also becoming more and more popular as acne sufferers find relief through the various applications of light.

It is well known that sunlight is good for clearing up acne, as long as you don't burn your skin in the process.

What has *not* always been understood is *why* light therapy benefits the skin.

What we consider to be just plain light is actually a spectrum of many different colored lights. Specifically, the blue and red wavelengths in sunlight are the ones that help the skin prevent and heal acne.

How? Each wavelength has a different length and effect. The red spectrum of light penetrates deeply into the skin.

When it does so, it activates hemoglobin and limits the blood supply to glands that produce oil.

This means less oil, which translates to fewer clogged pores and less acne.

Blue light is antibacterial – it penetrates into the skin's pores and kills much of the skin's acne-causing bacteria.

Both red and blue light therapies can be used, and are most effective if they are part of a total acne treatment regimen.

Light therapy is extremely flexible and doesn't have to be expensive. In fact, you can do blue or red spectrum light treatments in the privacy of your own homes, at the doctor's office or even at the spa.

Home light treatment systems start at around $100.00 USD up to hundreds of dollars. Some provide blue light, some red light, and some a combination of the two.

Be sure to check reviews and talk to your dermatologist before adding light therapy to your acne skin care regimen.

I personally bought a blue light therapy home machine for less than $100 from Amazon.

If you conduct a search on Amazon for "Blue Light Therapy", there home machines for less than $100.

You will need a course of 10 x 30min treatments, so purchasing a blue light therapy machine is well worth the investment.

Natural Remedies Action Plan

1. Select one or two of the listed above natural remedies and perform a treatment on yourself 2-3 times a week.

2. Before, during and after trying acne remedies, keep track of the effects in your acne journal. This will help you determine which remedies work best for your skin.

3. Blue Light therapy - Consider buying a blue light therapy machine second hand or from Amazon. These machines are well worth it and it gives you a chance to lie down and de-stress under blue light.

Prescription Acne Treatments

I left prescription acne treatments last as it should be your last resort. Like all prescription medications, there are without doubt negative side effects and may result in long term damage to your body so I would advise against it.

Prescription acne medications come in many different types, some are topical, and some are taken orally.

If your doctor or dermatologist prescribes one of these prescription-strength acne medications, it's important to understand exactly what they do.

10 Most Frequently Used Acne Medications

Below are ten of the most frequently used prescription acne medications today:

1. Isotretinoin (sold as: Accutane, Amesteem, Claravis and Sotret)
Isotretinoin is a powerful oral acne medication that is actually a form of vitamin A. It helps to resolve acne breakouts by limiting your oil glands production, and also helping your skin to renew itself more quickly. This can prevent dead skin cells and excess oils from clogging pores.

As stated before, isotretinoin is a very strong medication. When taking isotretinoin, you cannot donate blood or take additional vitamin A supplements in any form.

The most severe side effect of isotretinoin is actually its potential to cause life-threatening birth defects.

In fact, adolescent or adult women who are deemed to be of "child-bearing potential" must take pregnancy tests and agree in writing to use two forms of birth control while taking isotretinoin.

2. Tazarotene (Tazorac)

Tazorac is a vitamin A-based gel used for both acne and psoriasis. Unlike many acne treatment creams, tazarotene can be used alongside other acne topical treatments.

This medication works by limiting inflammation and reducing the number of clogged pores, and has shown promising effectiveness. In one study, an improvement of about fifty percent was seen after 12 weeks of use.

3. Tretinoin (Retin-A, Avita, Renova)

Tretinoin is a combination of retinoic acid and vitamin A, and is usually applied topically once a day.

This medication increases the rate at which skin cells are replaced to help keep pores and follicles clear. It also has been shown to reduce inflammation.

It shares many of the same potential side effects as other acne treatment gels or creams, such as redness, irritation and swelling of the skin.

4. Azelaic acid (Azelex)

Azelaic acid is believed to work in three different ways to help clear and prevent acne.

First, it helps to rejuvenate skin so that dead cell build up won't contribute to acne.

Secondly, it kills acne causing bacteria for a healthier overall environment on your skin.

And lastly, it acts as an anti-inflammatory, calming skin and reducing painful inflammation from acne flares.

Side effects with azelaic acid are not very common, with less than 5% of users reporting any side effects.

Those that did experience problems generally reported burning, itching and/or stinging.

For those with dark complexions, it might be best to go with a different acne medication: a few people have reported a skin lightening side effect, and this problem has not yet been thoroughly researched.

5. Low-dose birth control pills for women (Yaz, Estrostep, Ortho Tri-Cyclen)

Birth control pills are an often-prescribed treatment for adolescent acne in females, reducing the amount of testosterone in the body.

For some women, this can have a significant impact in the number of outbreaks they experience. In fact, studies show an average decrease in acne of thirty to sixty percent when birth control pills are taken.

However the downside here is that you're introducing synthetic hormones into your system which may cause negative side effects and hormonal imbalance.

6. Spironolactone (Aldactone)

Since the male hormone androgen, which occurs in males and females, is often a cause of acne, oral spironolactone is sometimes used to treat acne in women. The side effects can be troublesome, and include weakness and a lack of energy, unusual bleeding or a loss of appetite.

7. Clindamycin (Cleocin T, Clindaderm, Clindets)

This topical antibiotic can be prescribed in a number of forms: gel, lotion or foam. Generally, it should be applied twice a day.

The primary benefit of this topical clindamycin is its ability to kill P. Acnes, the bacteria that causes acne breakouts.

The most common negative side effects are all related to irritation of the skin, with burning, itching, redness and peeling at the top of the list. These side effect may appear at the start of treatment, and lessen after a few days.

8. Dapsone (Aczone)

Dapsone is generally prescribed in a 5% gel under the brand name Aczone. It deals primarily with the redness and irritation surrounding acne, and also acts as an antibacterial and antioxidant. Fortunately, the side effects that are associated with dapsone are mild, such as dryness and rash.

9. Erythromycin (Erygel, Akne-Mycin, Eryderm)

Erythromycin is a powerful topic antibiotic that is used to prevent skin infections and also minimize acne by killing the P. Acnes bacteria which causes it.

This antibiotic is often paired with benzoyl peroxide in prescription creams like Benzamycin. Side effects include burning, dryness, itching and redness.

Prescription Acne Action Plan

Talk to your doctor and conduct your own research - Remember acne prescription medication may provide relief but it is not a long term solution for curing acne. It's provided here as an option if you prefer to go the medical prescription route.

A Step By Step Radiant Skin Action Plan

As we've discussed throughout this book, there are many ways you can heal your acne. For some people, acne cures can happen on an external level while others focus on internal health.

I find that Acne is multi-factorial and the basic foundations in clearing acne FAST are:

- 10 to 20 minutes day for meditation or relaxation
- Vitamin supplementation
- Balance pH of skin & body

- Maintaining gut health i.e. probiotics
- A clean colorful diet comprising of vegetables, lean protein and healthy fats.
- Smart natural skin care regime
- Sweating it out with exercise and sauna

The strategies and remedies outline throughout this book has help cured my acne without resorting to prescription medications but there are no one-size-fits-all solutions to acne.

That's why it's up to you to do your own research, keep a daily journal and figure out what the main causes of your acne is so that you can develop your own acne cure plan that *specific to you.*

If you do so, do one small method at a time to see how your skin and body reacts.

A Step By Step Plan That Incorporates All The Best Options:

Step 1: Start an Acne Journal Today
Whether you keep your acne journal online or in a notebook, start tracking your acne today. Take note of your skin's current health, your water and food intake, whether or not you exercise, any medications you're on and your skin care regimen and whether or not you followed it.

Add anything else to your journal that you might think applies, such as your stress level; when it comes to tracking the causes of your acne, it's always better to have too much information than not enough.

Step 2: pH Balancing & Gut Health
Alkalize your skin, body and ensure that you have good bacteria to ensure your body's system is functioning properly. Look into pH facial cleansers, toners and consider using ACV to detox and cleanse your internal body. Follow this up with taking probiotics to maintain good gut health in order to reduce inflammation.

Step 3: Stay Hydrated
Whether you drink bottled water, juice or tea - ensure that they are not sugar laden beverages as proper hydration

can help to ensure optimum skin health. You should drink approximately nine cups of liquid if you're a woman, and thirteen if you're a man.

Step 4: Nutritious Diet That is Gluten & Dairy Free

Although no specific foods have been linked to acne outbreaks, studies have shown that people who eat diets low in monounsaturated fats have fewer problems with acne.

Consider taking a break from wheat and dairy for a short period to see if they are the cause of your acne.

Also, the vitamins and nutrients that come with a healthy diet can promote clear skin.

These include vitamin A, vitamin E, zinc and Omega-3 fatty acids (you can take it in the form of vitamin supplements).

Step 5: Create Your Own Healthy Skin Regimen – and Stick to It!

This means finding a pH balanced cleanser formulated for acne-prone skin and using it faithfully day and night. To further improve the pH of your skin, try adding a toner to your skin care regimen.

Definitely try a 4-6% niacinimide gel or serum and see if your skin clears up (it did for me!).

Spot creams like benzoyl peroxide or salicylic acid can be used to alleviate and treat problem areas.

Step 6: Manage Your Stress
Pay attention to your stress levels. When you start feeling too stressed out, take steps to reduce that stress, such as meditation and getting more sleep.

Step 7: Start Exercising Regularly
Whether you join a gym or simply jog around the neighborhood, an active lifestyle promotes overall health – which includes healthier skin! Just 20-30mins exercise improves blood flow to the skin, carrying nutrients and oxygen all over the body and removing impurities. Plus, exercise helps you sweat, which helps open and unclog pores.

Step 8: Consider a Sauna Regimen With Blue Light

Many people find that a proper sauna regimen can work wonders when it comes to clearing acne. Using a sauna at home or at your local gym and blue light therapy to heal your skin.

Step 9: Give Natural Remedies a Try

All ten of the natural remedies listed in Chapter 6 have worked for countless individuals. Although there's no telling if a specific natural remedy will work for you, it might – so give it a try!

Almost all of the natural remedies listed are low cost and easy to prepare, with no adverse side effects. As you try each natural remedy, keep careful notes in your acne journal of how you like it, and whether or not it worked for your skin.

Step 10: Talk to Your Doctor About Prescription Medications

If after 3 months, a great skin care regimen and an acne diet is not calming down your acne, talk to your doctor or dermatologist about the many prescription medications available to help acne sufferers.

<u>This should be your last resort.</u>

As with all prescription medications, there are side effects so please do your research first before you take any prescription medication (even if your doctor recommends it).

However I must stress that in the beginning, I did not nourish my body properly and use simple pH balance cleaners - I got lazy and preferred the "easy way" of getting a prescription.

After not getting the results I wanted, I then implemented the methods and strategies outlined in this book rigorously and stuck to it. After 3 months, my acne cleared.

Bonus - Acne Scar Treatments

A scar is formed as a part of the natural healing process of any wound or injury. When the skin layer or epidermis is damaged, the formation of scars happens. Acne scars are the result of inflamed skin lesions, cuts to the skin such as squeezing pimples.

Types of Acne Scars

Ice pick: This type of scar is deep, pitted, and usually two millimeters across or less. The appearance of the skin basically looks like it has been punctured with an ice pick, hence the name.

Boxcar: The scars have angular sharp edges and can sometimes look like scars from chicken pox. They can be shallow, deep, or sharp-edged and are found most often in the areas of the cheeks and temples.

Rolling: This type of scar is caused by damage under the skin's surface. They are most often wide and shallow, which gives the skin a wave-like appearance.

Hypertrophic: Hypertrophic scars most often appear on a person's chest and back. They are described as raised lumps and are a result of severe acne.

Side Note: Acne can leave reddish dark spots or marks on the skin after it heals. These marks are technically not scars but they occur due to hyper pigmentation of the skin and can last from 3-6 months. Hyper pigmentation can be easily addressed with natural remedies, which we will be covered later on.

Can acne scars be treated?

Yes, acne scars can be treated but the results will vary depending on the type of scarring and the method chosen for treatment.

Many acne scar treatments focus on fading the scar and making it less noticeable. It is important to understand that the scars itself cannot permanently removed unless the tissues that make up the scars are physically cut out or sloughed off.

Natural Scar Treatments

It is always a good idea to try natural home remedies to treat acne scars. First, the ingredients required are generally inexpensive and easy to find.

Second, side effects are very minimal or none at all. Acne and acne scars are a natural occurrence so it makes sense to treat them through natural ways as well.

Here are some acne scar remedies that are proven to reduce and treat scars:

Lemon Juice

The acidity of lemon juice makes it abrasive and able to strip away dead skin cells and old scar tissue. It acts like a mild chemical peel that allows the top layers of the skin to shed off to make way for newer skin cells.

The vitamin C is an added bonus, as it helps induce collagen production and assist in skin renewal. Lemon juice is also a natural bleaching agent that can help to lighten dark scars and make them less noticeable.

How it is applied:
- Squeeze some fresh lemon in clean bowl and use a cotton ball or swab to apply the juice on the acne scars.
- You have two options, you can let the juice sit on your skin for 10-15mins then rinse off with water or

- If you can withstand the sting, leave the lemon juice on your skin overnight before washing it off with lukewarm water.

Tips to remember:
- Lemon juice can cause irritation on sensitive skin. If this occurs, diluting the lemon juice with equal parts water before application can lessen the sting.
- Exposure to sunlight causes the lemon juice's bleaching properties to backfire. Instead of lightening, the lemon juice-soaked skin will darken, so always wear a hat and apply sunscreen when you head out.

Potato Juice

The humble potato is rich in skin rejuvenating nutrients such as phosphorus, sulfur, vitamin C, and potassium. The juice from potatoes has some bleaching properties that can help to fade scars.

How it is applied:
Rub sliced potato pieces on the skin areas with acne scars and leave on for twenty minutes before rinsing with cold water.

Tomato Pulp

Tomatoes has lycopene, which is an antioxidant that gives the tomato its vibrant red color. Lycopene helps boosts your immune system and aids in the production, growth, and regeneration of skin cells and appearance of skin texture.

It is also rich in vitamin A, which helps to improve skin appearance and help new skin tissues grow.

How it is applied:
- Create tomato pulp by dicing them and crushing them with the back of a spoon.
- Apply the pulp on the face, most especially on the scarred areas.
- Let the skin soak up the juices for one hour before washing with lukewarm water.

Tip to remember:
Do not use soap when washing off the pulp, as it can lessen the effect of the tomato juices.

Aloe Vera

Aloe vera flesh and juice is potent for skin healing; it contains saponin, a compound with anti-inflammatory, antibacterial, and anti-fungal properties that can lessen the reddish discoloration of acne scars. It will not only heal existing acne and prevent breakouts, but heal old acne scars as well!

How it is applied:
Extract the gel from the leaf of an aloe plant and apply directly on the scars caused by acne. Let the gel sit for an hour before rinsing and wiping the face. Applying the aloe vera gel twice daily can help to treat scarring.

Essential Oils

Oil based treatments help to moisturize the skin and is a natural alternative for treating mature acne scars. Some oils are thicker in consistency and may require dilution with carrier oils such as grape seed, sunflower, or apricot oil, before applying to the skin.

Used correctly, essential oils can loosen dead skin cells, promote better skin renewal, and fade acne scars. I'll point out the top essential oils that are commonly used to treat acne scars and will explain how to apply it.

Olive Oil: The moisturizing property of olive oil improves skin texture by making it soft and supple. This makes acne scars less apparent.

Rose-hip Seed Oil: This oil has anti-aging properties and is used in various cosmetic products to treat acne scarring. It helps to regenerate the skin and lessens discoloration.

Lavender Oil: Lavender oil has some regenerative properties that revitalize the skin and help to treat acne scars.

Coconut Oil: Apart from moisturizing, coconut oil also contains nutrients that are good for the skin. It has vitamin E, lauric acid, and capric acid.

Tea Tree Oil: It is moisturizing and has anti-inflammatory properties as well. It helps to remove impurities and promotes skin healing.

How it is applied: Warm the chosen oil slightly and apply directly on the acne scar. Massage lightly with your fingers or a cotton bud for 5 minutes on your scar and wipe off excess oil.

Tip to remember: The oil to be applied should be as warm as your own body temperature. Oil that is too hot will burn the skin and cause further damage.

Cucumber

The high water content hydrates the skin and keeps it cool, which reduces the inflammation and redness associated with scarring. Cucumbers can tone, calm, reduce puffiness and lighten scars.

How it is applied:
Mash up a cucumber (skin and juice) and regularly apply it to your acne scars, you should see an improvement within just a few days. For best results, apply daily and consistently.

Green Papaya

Green, unripe papaya is full of Alpha Hydroxy Acids (AHA's), which help lighten skin pigmentation left from acne, decrease the appearance of fine lines and wrinkles, and treat sun damaged skin. This fruit contains an enzyme called papain, which acts as a natural skin exfoliant that helps skin cells to renew faster.

How it is applied:

Cut up papaya slices, blend it in a food mixer, and apply as a mask directly on the acne scars for about 10 minutes before washing off with water.

Tips to remember:

- If any irritation is noticed, remove the papaya slice from the skin immediately.

- The application should not last more than fifteen minutes, as the papaya slices can leave the skin red, raw, and painful.

Orange Peels

Orange peels are rich in retinol, which encourages natural skin exfoliation. It also stimulates collagen production, which helps to rebuild and repair skin cells.

How it is applied:
Dried orange peel powder can be mixed with milk and applied on the skin, or it can be added to rosewater and applied as well.

Fenugreek Extract

It has anti-inflammatory properties that can heal eczema, burns, and boils.

Grounded fenugreek seeds along with water can greatly reduce the appearance of acne scars.

How it is applied:
- Boil five milliliters of fenugreek seeds in two hundred fifty milliliters of water for ten to fifteen minutes.
- Allow to cool before straining the seeds and applying to the acne scars.
- Do not rinse off the solution.
- Repeat the application daily for one week.

Neem Leaves

These have alkaloids that have antibacterial and antiviral properties which help to clean acne affected areas and promote natural healing.

How it is applied:

Place a neem leaf directly on acne scars and hold in place for about fifteen minutes. Repeat the application daily for about one week or longer if necessary.

Tip: If you can't find fresh neem leaves, head to an Indian grocery store and purchase pure neem powder, mix into a paste, and apply directly on your scars.

Egg Whites

The protein and amino acids in egg whites can help to speed up the healing process of the skin and boost up acne scar recovery.

How it is applied:

Apply the egg whites on the acne scars with the use of a cotton ball or swab and leave on overnight. Rinse with water after.

Turmeric

Turmeric has long been known in the West as a spice that adds flavor and color to Indian dishes or as an Ayurveda or Chinese medicine.

In many parts of India, turmeric is an essential part of any beauty treatment. When applied to the skin as a paste or a face mask, it can help in treating acne, acne scars, eczema, rosacea, and aids in skin rejuvenation.

How it is applied:
Turmeric can be added to food and ingested, or made into a paste by adding a few drops of water to turmeric powder.

The paste is the applied to the scars and left on for 10-15 minutes before washing off.

Honey

It has antibacterial properties and is rich in minerals such as magnesium, potassium, calcium, sodium chlorine, sulfur, and iron that promote growth of skin tissue.

How it is applied:

Massage or rub organic raw honey on acne scars for 5 minutes twice daily and wash it off with cold water.

Fuller's Earth

This traditional clay material is great for absorbing oil, grease, and toxins from your skin. It can be used to clear out blocked skin pores, to treat oily skin, and to diminish acne scars.

How it is applied:

The usual preparation is a fuller's earth powder face pack mixed with some rose water.

It is then applied directly to the skin and washed off after several minutes.

Curds

Curds are high in lactic acid, which is a mild bleaching agent. It can be used instead of citric acid (found in lemon juice and orange peels) and is best for those with sensitive skin. Also, the fat content in the curds act as a very good natural skin moisturizer.

Coconut Water

Directly applying coconut water on the skin helps to remove dead cells. This makes the skin brighter and acne scars less visible.

Sandalwood

Sandalwood has cooling properties that can soothe inflamed and irritated acne scars. It helps to speed up the skin's healing process.

How it is applied:
- Make a paste from sandalwood and rosewater and apply on the scarred areas of the face.
- Let the paste sit for an hour or overnight if possible before washing it off with cold water.
- Repeat the procedure at least once daily.

- Make sandalwood water by soaking a piece of sandalwood in water for a few hours.
- Dab the water on the acne scars with a cotton ball or swab.
- The procedure can be done on a daily basis.

Natural Skin Exfoliants

Sugar: Granulated sugar can be mixed with water to form an exfoliating paste that can gently slough away dead skin cells and strip away scar tissues.

How it is applied: Mix fifteen milliliters of granulated sugar with five to ten milliliters of water. Gently massage the paste with a circular motion on the entire face, focusing on the scarred areas. Wash off the scrub with warm water.

Besan or Gram Flour: Using besan as an exfoliating agent will help to reduce scars and brighten the skin. Sloughing away the dead skin cells will make way for the growth of new ones.

How it is applied: Mix besan with water to make a paste that can be used as a facial scrub.

Oatmeal: Besides exfoliation, oatmeal can also help to soothe irritated and inflamed skin. Mixing it with water and applying it to the face can help to remove dead skin cells and old scar tissue.

How it is applied: Combine ten milliliters of oatmeal with the same amount of water. Massage gently on the face in a circular motion and let the mixture sit for five minutes before washing off with warm water.

Apple Cider Vinegar: Vinegar has abrasive properties that make it effective in removing dead skin cells. It is also a natural antiseptic which can further help in the skin's healing and renewal processes.

How it is applied: Combine same amounts of apple cider vinegar and water. Dab the solution on the acne scars with the use of cotton balls or swabs. Let it sit for a few hours before washing off with lukewarm water.

Tip to remember: Buy apple cider vinegar with mother (i.e. cloudy vinegar) but remember that vinegar is a very harsh substance. Avoid applying undiluted vinegar onto the skin, as this can cause irritation, especially on sensitive skin.

Baking Soda: When baking soda is mixed with water, it can help to unclog facial pores and strip away old skin cells and bacteria as well. This promotes the formation of newer cells and the renewal of the skin in general.

How it is applied: Make a paste by mixing fifteen milliliters of baking soda and five milliliters of water. More of either ingredient can be added to prevent it from being too runny or watery. Apply the baking powder paste on the acne scars and let it sit for about two to three minutes. Wash the face and rinse the paste off with lukewarm water. This procedure can be done twice daily.

Choosing Acne Scar Treatment Products

There are a variety of over the counter products that can be used to treat acne scars. The main problem is choosing the right one. Think of what you want to achieve and start from there.

One trick to finding products that are effective is to pay attention to the ingredients. Knowing what the components are and what they do can help to determine if they can have a significant effect on acne scars.

Sunscreen

Sunlight can further darken scars and slow down the skin's healing process. Ultraviolet rays stimulate pigment production, which can lead to discoloration.

Tips to remember:
- Apply sunscreen twenty minutes before going outdoors.
- Choose preparations that are oil free to prevent future acne breakouts. Labels to look out for include: oil-free, won't clog pores, and non-comedogenic.
- Look for products that have a sun protection factor of thirty or higher. These days, sunscreens have an SPF of 50+, so the higher the better.
- Choose those labeled as broad spectrum. This kind of sunscreen is able to protect the skin from ultraviolet A and ultraviolet B rays.

Silicone gels, sheets, dressings, and bandages

These are used for healing closed wounds and to reduce inflammation. They help to minimize the occurrence of keloids and hypertrophic or raised scars.

Tip to remember:
To achieve the best results, the silicone gels are placed on the scar for twelve hours every day for at least three months.

Ingredients to Look Out For In Over the Counter Products

Kojic Acid: This is a natural skin lightening substance that is derived from mushroom extracts. It is a usual ingredient in lotions, creams, and soaps.

Retinol: This substance helps to prevent skin pores from being blocked and clogged. It helps to clear the skin from old cells and gives way for the production of new ones.

Alpha Hydroxy Acids: These substances act as exfoliants. They act on the cells of the epidermis, making it easier for dead skin cells to be sloughed off. This promotes re-growth of new skin cells. They can also stimulate the production of collagen and elastin, which are important in keeping good skin integrity.

The five major types of alpha hydroxyl acids used in skin care products are:

- **Glycolic Acid:** It is usually extracted from sugarcane,

unripe grapes, pineapple, and melons.
- **Ascorbic Acid:** This is otherwise known as Vitamin C. As was previously mentioned, it helps in collagen production and skin renewal.
- **Lactic Acid:** Found in milk and other dairy products
- **Malic Acid:** Extracted from apples and pears
- **Tartaric Acid:** Primarily found in grapes

Corticosteroids: Topical cortisone creams can help to minimize any kind of scarring. The cream is usually applied once or twice daily. Take note, as this type of cream can dry out the skin, so it is ideally used along with a skin moisturizer.

Sun exposure is also minimized, as the cortisone can make the skin more sensitive to sunlight. The side effects of this treatment include: thinning of the skin, stretch marks, easy bruising, and skin tearing.

Side Note: Hydroquinone is a popular whitening agent that is a cause for concern, as studies have shown that it can be potentially carcinogenic.

Tips to Remember:
- Test the products on a small area of your skin before purchasing anything. Every person's reaction to any substance is unique. Some may cause allergic or sensitivity reactions while others may not.

- Put a small amount of the product on the inner area of you arm or behind your ear. If there is no reaction, such as redness, itching, swelling, and burning sensations, then the product is safe to use.
- The effectiveness of treatments for acne scars is also dependent on skin color, skin thickness, and individual skin structure.
- Consistency is the key to achieving the best results. Jumping from one product to another will not do the skin any good.
- It takes some time for a specific product to have any effect. Regular application will allow the medication to adequately penetrate the skin and take its

proper effect.

When in doubt, it is always a good idea to consult dermatological experts and practitioners. Options can be discussed before settling on a specific choice.

Learn to read labels and familiarize yourself with words and ingredients that are important enough to take note of.

Professional Scar Removal Treatments

When home remedies are not effective and when scarring is extensive, seeking the help from dermatologists and skin doctors can stop the inflammatory process that results in scarring and provides faster results.

Depending on the skin's condition and the extent of tissue damage, a combination of different professional treatments using medical devices are typically required to achieve satisfactory results.

There are several options available for acne scar removal and each technique carries different risks, so be sure to discuss potential side effects and results with your chosen practitioner.

Here are some professional acne scar removal treatments you can look into:

Microdermabrasion

This method involves the removal of the skin's topmost layer. This is achieved with the use of a rapidly rotating wire brush. This procedure is most appropriate for superficial scars. Pitted and deep scars are not completely removed but are made to appear less noticeable.

Chemical Peels

A mixture of chemicals is applied to the face to make the skin's upper layer peel off. Scarring can be reduced and skin discoloration is treated as well.

Skin Needling

Skin needling is a procedure that involves puncturing the skin multiple times with small sterilized needles attached to a cylindrical roller (called a derma roller).

The needles cause thousands of micro-injuries to the skin, which induces collagen growth and improves the appearance of acne scars.

Better results can be achieved with a derma pen instead of a derma roller, as the derma pen comes with an electric motor and allows for even skin needling with less down time.

Injectable Fillers

Fillers containing hyaluronic acid or your own autologous fat (which involves harvesting fat from thighs or stomach) can be injected into the atrophic scars.

Injectable fillers containing hyaluronic acid only last 6-12 months, whilst autologous fat injections may last several years. The lack of permanence and cost of repeat visits makes this option less popular.

Ablative Resurfacing

A wounding (ablative) laser sends energy pulses to remove thin layers of your skin, typically involving the use of carbon dioxide CO_2 and erbium.

The downtime is usually 2 weeks and be warned, you will look like you've been burnt, however you can expect a 50% improvement in scar correction from just 2-3 ablative laser treatments.

Non Ablative Resurfacing

Non ablative lasers are a non-wounding laser, which stimulates collagen growth and tightens underlying skin.

Although non-ablative laser resurfacing is less invasive and requires less recovery time, it's less effective than is ablative laser resurfacing. You may require 5 to 10 treatments before you notice a moderate improvement in acne scars.

Factional CO2 Resurfacing

Fractional Carbon dioxide lasers can be used to resurface skin, remove sun damage and acne scars, and tighten skin on the face.

They work by removing a fine layer of skin, as well as heating the skin. This remodels the skin's collagen, and leads to significantly smoother, firmer, and more even toned skin.

Despite the dramatic results, there are many downsides to treatment with traditional carbon dioxide lasers. The risks of traditional carbon dioxide laser treatment include prolonged recovery periods, gradual loss of skin pigmentation, and a relatively high risk of scarring if performed incorrectly by an unskilled surgeon.

Combination Treatments

A combination treatment that involves using tumescent anesthesia, extensive subcision, chemical peeling, laser resurfacing, and fraxel repair laser treatment can result in 80% improvement in acne scars.

Speak to a cosmetic doctor to see if he has a similar scar removal treatment package. Downtime is 7-14days.

Surgery

Deep acne scars can be treated by punch grafts, punch excisions, and subcision. This is where individual acne scars are cut out and the hole that is left is either sutured closed or repaired with a skin graft.

Tissue Fillers

This method involves directly injecting collagen under the skin's surface to fill out the cavities caused by scars or to stretch out the skin and make the acne scars less visible. The injections are usually repeated as the results are temporary.

Corticosteroid Injections

This procedure is primarily used for keloid and hypertrophic scars. A series of injections are made into the raised scar tissue to reduce inflammation.

The resulting effect is a flattened scar. The scar is not removed but the appearance is improved. Depending on the scar, the procedure is repeated over several months.

Corticosteroid injections are given three times at four to six week intervals to assess for body response and scar tissue improvement.

The downside is that it's costly, and from my personal experience with keloid scars, after going through corticosteroid injection was using plain, simple tea tree oil.

Apply tea tree oil with a cotton bud; massage the keloid for 20 minutes before bed time. You will notice the lump softening within 2 weeks and scabbing in which new skin is revealed.

Radio Frequency (RF) Treatments

This method of scar revision does not use laser light but uses radio frequency energy to remodel collagen and scars.

The pulse of energy is delivered via a fractional technique into the deeper layers of skin. Energy and heat breaks down the scar tissue, with minimal damage to the upper layers of skin.

This process is gentle, and has very little, if any, downtime. RF can be used as a stand-alone treatment for acne scars or combined with non ablative laser treatments.

Acne Scar Tips and Tricks

1. Prevention is more effective than cure. This statement may seem a bit glib, but there is no denying the truth to it. The most effective way to get rid of acne scars is to not develop them. Acne formation can be prevented and if they are already present, scar formation can be avoided by improving the whole healing process.

2. Use makeup for cosmetic camouflage. If any of the acne scar treatments do not work, then using makeup to cover them up is effective. Although the effect is temporary, makeup is particularly useful for acne scars on the face. There are specially manufactured products that are meant to cover up blemishes and scarring. These are readily available over the counter in most pharmacies. Color matching can be performed by qualified personnel to achieve the best results.

3. Be careful with commercially produced abrasive facial or body scrubs. Scrubs that are too hard and too abrasive can aggravate existing scarring and can cause new scars to develop.

4. Squeezing pimples can cause acne scars. Yes, it may be tempting but please don't squeeze your pimples, the squeezing action itself can cause tissue damage around the pores or follicles. Furthermore, your nails may contain bacteria and cause pus and other toxic material in the pimple to damage the skin's natural collagen.

That's a wrap! I hope you enjoyed the Radiant Skin - Acne Treatment Book.

Remember - Don't Give Up!

Curing your acne isn't just one thing that you do. For most of us who deal with acne outbreaks, it's a process.

The most important step in any journey is always the first one, and you are taking ten important steps when you begin the program I've outlined above.

If one step doesn't have an immediate impact, keep trying, track your progress and never stop working towards clear, comfortable skin!

Take care
Aimee xx

Free Gift

Get your FREE "Radiant Skin - Beat Acne Checklist"

Print out this DAILY checklist with step by step instructions on what you should do in the morning, afternoon and night to help you beat acne!

Get your FREE "Acne Checklist" at:

Goo.gl/b9n1mw

Other Books By Aimee

HEALTH & BEAUTY SERIES

Book 1:
ACNE TREATMENT BOOK - The Adult Acne Treatment Book With Proven Acne Remedies & Treatments To Cure Cystic & Hormonal Acne For Radiant Skin

Book 2:
VOGUE HACK - The 3 Step Intermittent Fasting System To Lose Up To 10 Pounds In 10 Days & Achieve Rapid Fat Loss.

Book 3:
10 YEARS YOUNGER - Look Younger With Yoga Face Exercises, Get Rid of

Wrinkles & Take 10 Years off Your Face in 8 Mins A Day.

Book 4:

CELLULITE BLASTER - Quick Start Guide To Getting Rid Of Cellulite FAST and Blasting Them Off Your Stomach, Thighs, Legs & Butt!

You can simply search for "Aimee Blake" on the Amazon Kindle store or visit my author page at: **Amazon.com/Aimee-Blake/e/ B0754JR3M4**

About The Author

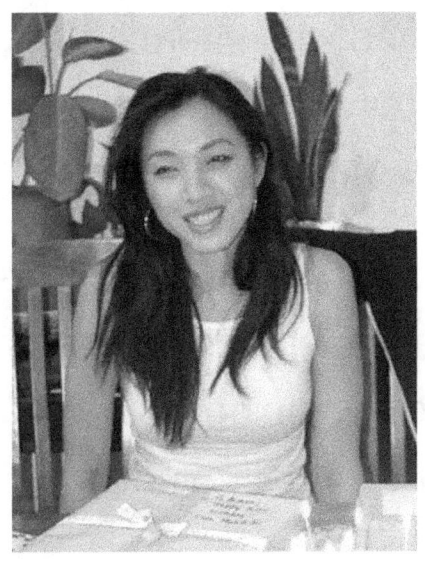

Aimee Blake is from Sydney Australia - she's a self experimenter of all things health, beauty and wellness and is a certified nutritionist.

In October 2013, she lost over 25 pounds in less than 2.5 months without restrictive diets, cardio whilst still eating the foods she loves!

This led her to writing "Vogue Hack" - a simple 3 step weight loss system that helps women with intermittent fasting, losing 10 pounds in 10 days and dropping a dress size fast!

She's written books on skin care and natural anti aging solutions and is committed to helping women all over the world improve their mind, body and spirit.

Thank You… And One Tiny Favor, Please

Thank you for reading my book! I really value your feedback and would appreciate it if you could leave a review.

As an independent author, I have a heart for helping people by sharing the information presented in this book.

Please leave me a helpful review on Amazon right now by turning to the last page and leave a 5 star rating as it will help others have confidence in buying the book.

It would really help benefit other people and Zeus my doggy values your opinion as well!

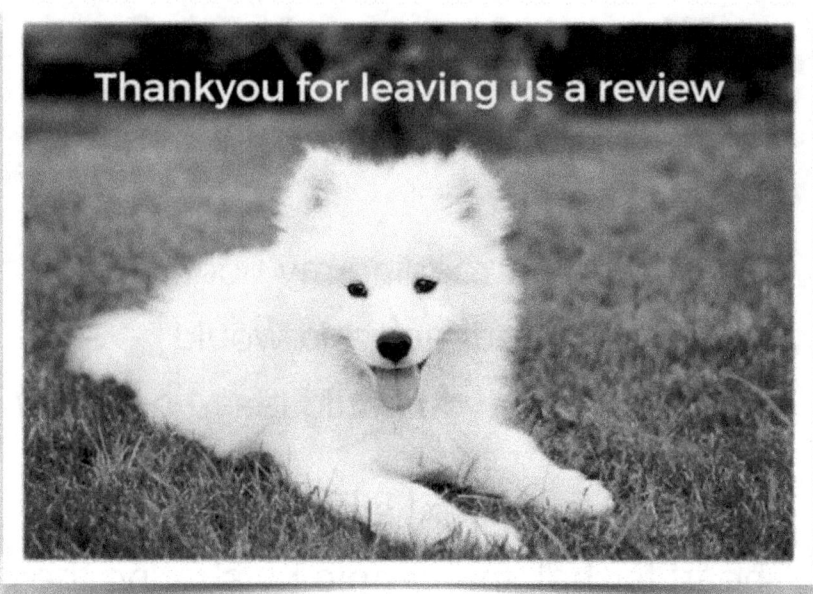